The DASH DIET MEAL PREP

Delicious Heart-Healthy Recipes Low-Sodium, High-Potassium to Manage Blood Pressure

Adam C.

ISBN: 9798872905271

DEDICATION

This book is dedicated to all my Readers

CONTENTS

Chapter 1: Introduction

1.1 Understanding the DASH Diet

Welcome to "The DASH DIET MEAL PREP: Delicious Heart-Healthy Recipes Low-Sodium, High-Potassium to Manage Blood Pressure." In this chapter, we will embark on a journey to understand the DASH (Dietary Approaches to Stop Hypertension) Diet a dietary approach renowned for its effectiveness in managing blood pressure and promoting overall cardiovascular health.

The DASH Diet's History

In the 1990s, the National Heart, Lung, and Blood Institute (NHLBI) supported innovative research that resulted in the development of the DASH Diet. A food plan that is specifically intended to decrease and control blood pressure without the need for medication was developed through collaboration between scientists and nutrition professionals. This nutritional strategy places an emphasis on a balance of nutrients, with a specific goal of lowering sodium consumption.

Fundamental Ideas of the DASH Diet

The DASH Diet is based on several important ideas that support heart health and general well-being:

1. Increased Fruit and Vegetable Intake: Fruits and vegetables are a key component of the DASH Diet since they are full of important vitamins, minerals, and antioxidants. These foods are high in nutrients and can reduce the risk of cardiovascular illnesses.

2. Focus on Whole Grains: The fiber found in whole grains contributes to the maintenance of good cholesterol levels. Whole grains are substituted for refined grains in the DASH Diet in order to improve nutritional value and promote heart health.

3. Lean Protein Sources: Fish, poultry, legumes, nuts, and seeds are examples of lean protein sources that are recommended by the diet. These choices promote cardiovascular health by providing protein without the saturated fats present in some red meats.

4. Low-Fat Dairy Products: While dairy products are allowed under the DASH Diet, low-fat or fat-free varieties are the main focus. These supply vital nutrients without having too many saturated fats.

5. Limited Sodium Intake: Cutting back on sodium is one of the main tenets of the DASH Diet. The diet lowers blood pressure and lowers the risk of consequences from hypertension by consuming less salt.

1.2 Importance of Meal Prep for Health

The DASH Diet requires proper meal preparation in order to be successfully followed. It might be difficult to find the time to cook heart-healthy, balanced meals as our lives get busier. Meal prep helps us to fill the gap between our hectic schedules and our dedication to good health in this situation.

1. Time-Saving Convenience: Meal prep helps you save time during the week by planning and cooking meals ahead of time. You can guarantee that wholesome meals that adhere to the DASH Diet are always available by creating meticulous meal plans and planning ahead for meal preparation.

2. Portion Control and Nutrient Balance: Meal preparation gives you the ability to manage portion sizes and guarantee that nutrients are distributed in a balanced manner. You can control ingredient amounts when you cook at home, which will help you stick to the daily allowance of fruits, vegetables, whole grains, and lean proteins.

3. Reducing the Temptation of Unhealthy Options: The temptation to choose fast food or unhealthy snacks is lessened when meals are prepared and waiting. Meal preparation puts you in a successful position by removing the need for impulsive, unhealthy food decisions.

4. Long-Term Success and Consistency: The success of any diet plan depends on consistency. Making DASH Diet-compliant meals on a regular basis helps you create a pattern that promotes your long-term health objectives. A sustainable and doable strategy to leading a heart-healthy lifestyle is fostered by meal prep.

1.3 Benefits of the DASH Diet for Blood Pressure Management

1. Scientifically Proven Blood Pressure Reduction: The DASH Diet has been shown in numerous clinical studies to be effective in lowering blood pressure. A focus on foods high in potassium and a decrease in sodium intake lead to better cardiovascular health and blood vessel function.

2. Reduced Risk of Hypertension: The DASH Diet is useful in lowering the risk of developing high blood pressure as well as for individuals who already have hypertension. Its focus on a diet rich in nutrients and well-balanced encourages the best possible cardiovascular health.

3. Comprehensive Heart Health: The DASH Diet tackles several facets of heart health in addition to blood pressure control. Incorporating fruits, vegetables, whole grains, and lean meats promotes cardiovascular health by lowering inflammation and maintaining healthy cholesterol levels.

5. Weight Management Support: The DASH Diet's emphasis on whole, nutrient-dense foods naturally helps with weight control, even though it was not created as a weight-loss plan. Fostering a healthy eating pattern lowers the risk factors linked to cardiovascular illnesses and encourages weight loss or maintenance that is sustainable.

As we go deeper into "The DASH DIET MEAL PREP," each chapter will walk you through doable tactics, mouthwatering dishes, and useful advice on incorporating the DASH Diet into your daily routine. Prepare yourself for a delicious and heart-healthy trip that will change the way you think about food and wellness.

Chapter 2: Getting Started with DASH Diet Meal Prep

Welcome to the practical and hands-on chapter of "The DASH DIET MEAL PREP: Delicious Heart-Healthy Recipes Low-Sodium, High-Potassium to Manage Blood Pressure." This chapter will serve as your guide to setting up your kitchen, understanding essential tools and ingredients, and mastering the art of planning your DASH Diet meal prep.

2.1 Setting up Your Kitchen

The first step to easily incorporate heart-healthy meals into your routine is to make your kitchen DASH Diet compatible. Let's examine the essential components of a successful kitchen setup:

1. Organize Your Pantry:

- **Whole Grains:** Make sure you eat plenty of whole grains, such as whole wheat pasta, quinoa, brown rice, and oats. These serve as the basis for a lot of DASH Diet meals.
- **Canned Goods**: Choose tomatoes, beans, and veggies that are low in salt. These are easy pantry staples that will help you prepare wholesome meals quickly.

- **Healthy Oils:** For cooking and dressings, choose heart-healthy oils like canola and olive oil.

- **Herbs and Spices**: Use a range of herbs and spices to enhance flavor without adding extra salt. Think about alternatives such as cumin, garlic powder, oregano, and basil.

2. Prioritize Fresh Produce:

- **Colorful Vegetables:** To add color and nutrients to your meals, keep a variety of fresh veggies on hand, such as broccoli, bell peppers, carrots, and leafy greens.

- **Vibrant Fruits:** Keep a variety of fresh fruits on available for meals and snacks, such as bananas, apples, berries, and oranges.

3. Choose Lean Proteins:

- **Fish and Poultry:** Choose lean protein sources like skinless chicken breasts and a variety of fish options like tilapia and salmon.

- **Plant-Based Proteins:** For diversity and heart-healthy advantages, include plant-based proteins such beans, lentils, and tofu in your meals.

4. Upgrade Your Refrigerator and Freezer:

- **Low-Fat Dairy:** Keep an abundance of fat-free or low-fat dairy products on hand, including cheese, yogurt, and milk.
- **Frozen Vegetables:** To make quick and simple meal additions, keep a variety of frozen vegetables in your freezer.

5. Invest in DASH Diet-Friendly Snacks:

- **Nuts and Seeds:** For snacking and added nutritional value, include a variety of nuts and seeds, such as almonds, walnuts, chia seeds, and flaxseeds.
- **Greek Yogurt:** For a flexible and high-protein snack, go for plain, fat-free Greek yogurt.

2.2 Essential Tools and Ingredients

Equipping yourself with the necessary tools and ingredients is essential to an efficient and pleasurable DASH Diet meal prep. Let's examine the fundamentals:

1. Kitchen Tools:

- **Cutting Boards and Knives:** For effective and secure food preparation, make an investment in high-quality cutting boards and sharp blades.

- **Measuring Cups and Spoons:** For balanced nutrition and portion control, precise measurements are crucial.

- **Mixing Bowls:** A variety of sizes of mixing bowls come in helpful while blending ingredients and getting the components of several recipes ready.

- **Food Storage Containers:** Purchase a range of containers to keep prepared foods and meals fresh. To guarantee food safety, use glass or BPA-free plastic containers.

2. Cooking Appliances:

- **Quality Pots and Pans:** Purchase an assortment of pots and pans to suit various cooking methods, such as boiling and sautéing.

- **Slow Cooker or Instant Pot:** Slow cookers and instant pots are great time-savers for making stews and large quantities of food.

- **Blender or Food Processor:** A blender or food processor is necessary to quickly and easily make sauces, soups, and smoothies.

3. DASH Diet-Friendly Ingredients:

- **Low-Sodium Broths:** As a foundation for soups and stews, use low-sodium chicken or vegetable broth.

- **Whole Grain Flour:** Try baking using whole grain flours such as almond or whole wheat flour.

- **Low-Sodium Condiments:** To add flavor to your food without adding too much salt, use low-sodium mustard, vinegar, and soy sauce.

2.3 Planning Your DASH Diet Meal Prep

Effective meal preparation is essential to a successful DASH Diet. To make the process of getting ready go more smoothly, do these steps:

1. Set Realistic Goals:

- **Start Small:** If you've never prepared meals before, start with just one or two a week. You can work your way up to preparing for the full week as you get more accustomed to it.

- **Consider Your Schedule:** Match the days you are busiest with the times you prepare meals. Meal planning helps you have wholesome options on hand for those busy days.

2. Choose DASH Diet Recipes:

- **Explore Variety:** Choose a variety of DASH Diet dishes to add interest and enjoyment to your meals.
- **Consider Batch Cooking:** Select recipes that work well for large quantities of cooking. Casseroles, stews, and soups are great ways to make several servings at once.

3. Create a Meal Prep Calendar:

- **Designate Prep Days:** Determine which days, given your schedule, to prepare meals. For most people, Sunday and Wednesday are the best days to cook for the next week.
- **Map out Meals:** Make a weekly food plan that takes into account breakfast, lunch, dinner, and snacks. This guarantees balanced nourishment and assists you in making a thorough shopping list.

4. Efficient Shopping:

- **Follow Your List:** Adhere to your pre-made shopping list to prevent impulsive buys and maintain financial discipline.
- **Prioritize Fresh Produce:** To preserve freshness, purchase perishable goods closer to your prep days.

5. Batch Prep Ingredients:

- **Chop Vegetables:** Vegetables should be pre-chopped and kept in portioned containers for convenient access.
- **Prepare Proteins:** To incorporate into different dishes, cook proteins in quantity, such as roasted tofu or grilled chicken.
- **Portion Control:** Divide components such as grains, beans, and other items into portions based on your meal plan by using measurement tools.

6. Storage and Labeling:

- **Use Clear Containers:** To make it easier to recognize the contents and keep an eye on freshness, choose clear containers.
- **Label Containers:** To monitor freshness and prevent food waste, mark containers with the preparation date.

7. Stay Flexible:

- **Adapt as Needed:** Be willing to modify your meal preparation schedule in response to your changing needs, tastes, and dietary objectives.
- **Rotate Recipes:** To keep mealtime monotony at bay, periodically rotate in different recipes.

By preparing your kitchen, assembling the necessary equipment and supplies, and organizing your DASH Diet meal prep, you've established the foundation for an effective and long-lasting strategy for heart-healthy eating. We'll go into more detail on certain DASH Diet dishes and inventive methods to make meal planning fun and a regular part of your life in the next chapters. Prepare to taste the flavors of well-being and wellness!

Chapter 3: DASH Diet Fundamentals

Welcome to the heart of "The DASH DIET MEAL PREP: Delicious Heart-Healthy Recipes Low-Sodium, High-Potassium to Manage Blood Pressure." We shall examine the basic tenets of the DASH (Dietary Approaches to Stop Hypertension) Diet in this chapter. Achieving optimal heart health requires understanding the guidelines, modifying the diet to suit your needs, and including foods high in potassium and low in salt.

3.1 Overview of the DASH Diet Guidelines

A dietary strategy created especially to prevent and treat hypertension (high blood pressure) is the DASH Diet. Its cornerstone is the encouragement of a nutrient-rich, well-balanced diet. Let's examine the main rules that constitute the DASH Diet's framework:

1. Emphasis on Fruits and Vegetables:

- **Recommendation:** Aim to consume a variety of fruits and vegetables each day.

- **Benefits:** Fruits and vegetables are high in fiber, potassium, and magnesium, all of which help to control blood pressure. They also supply important antioxidants and vitamins for general wellness.

2. Whole Grains as a Staple:

- **Recommendation:** It is advised to select whole grains rather than refined grains.
- **Benefits:** Whole grains are a great source of fiber and other nutrients. Examples of these are brown rice, quinoa, and oats. They aid in the regulation of cholesterol levels, which promotes heart health.

3. Lean Protein Sources:

- **Recommendation:** Opt for lean protein sources such as poultry, fish, beans, nuts, and seeds.
- **Benefits:** Lean meats don't have the saturated fats that other red meats do, but they still deliver important amino acids. They promote cardiovascular health in general and muscle health in particular.

4. Low-Fat Dairy Products:

- **Recommendation:** It is advised to select dairy products that are either fat-free or low-fat.

- **Benefits:** Dairy products low in fat offer calcium, vitamin D, and other important nutrients without having too much saturated fat. They promote bone health and help maintain a balanced diet.

5. Limited Sodium Intake:

- **Recommendation**: Cut back on sodium by consuming fewer high-sodium foods and utilizing less additional salt.
- **Benefits:** Reducing salt consumption is essential for blood pressure management. The DASH Diet's main component is salt reduction because too much sodium can lead to blood pressure rise and fluid retention.

6. Moderation in Sweets and Added Sugars:

- **Recommendation**: Restrict your intake of added sugars and sweets.
- **Benefits**: The DASH Diet helps regulate calorie intake and promotes weight management by lowering the consumption of sugary foods and beverages.

7. Portion Control:

- **Recommendation:** Be mindful of portion sizes to avoid overeating.
- **Benefits:** Maintaining a healthy weight and overall nutritional balance depend on portion control. It

guarantees that you get the proper amount of nutrients without consuming too many calories.

8. Alcohol in Moderation:

- **Recommendation:** If you choose to consume alcohol, do so in moderation.
- **Benefits:** Red wine in particular has been linked to reduced alcohol intake's positive effects on the heart. But in order to prevent any unfavorable consequences, moderation is essential.

9. Balanced Macronutrient Distribution:

- **Recommendation:** In your everyday diet, strive for a balance between carbohydrates, proteins, and fats.
- **Benefits:** The distribution of macronutrients in a balanced way promotes energy metabolism and general health. It makes sure your body gets all the different kinds of nutrients it needs to function at its best.

10. Flexibility and Long-Term Adherence:

- **Recommendation:** Adapt the DASH Diet to your preferences and lifestyle for sustainable adherence.
- **Benefits:** The DASH Diet is adaptable and may be tailored to meet dietary constraints, cultural factors, and

personal preferences. This flexibility improves success and adherence over the long run.

3.2 Customizing the DASH Diet for Your Needs

Although the DASH Diet offers a good foundation for heart-healthy eating, it must be customized in order to become a sustainable and pleasurable aspect of your daily. To customize the DASH Diet to your specific needs, take into account the following strategies:

1. Identify Personal Preferences:

- **Favorite Foods:** List the fruits, vegetables, grains, and proteins that you prefer. Add these to your DASH Diet meals to increase your level of satisfaction.
- **Cultural Influences:** Think about the meals that are important to you and your cultural heritage. Look for methods to incorporate the DASH Diet's tenets into meals that suit your ethnic tastes.

2. Gradual Adjustments:

- **Slow Transition:** If the DASH Diet is a big change from your usual eating routine, think about implementing the changes gradually. One or two DASH-friendly meals a day is a good place to start, and you can increase this over time.

3. Experiment with Recipes:

- **Explore Variety:** Try out a range of DASH Diet dishes to find combinations and flavors that you like. A vast array of culinary discovery is made possible by the diversity of the diet.
- **Modify Recipes:** Feel free to adjust recipes to your personal preferences. Get inventive in the kitchen, change up the ingredients, and adjust the seasonings.

4. Seek Professional Guidance:

- **Consult a Nutritionist:** See a trained dietitian or nutritionist if you have any specific dietary questions or health issues. They may offer tailored advice and guarantee that the DASH Diet is in line with your particular health objectives.

5. Make Sustainable Changes:

- **Lifestyle Integration:** Integrating the DASH Diet's concepts into your lifestyle should be done in a way that works for you. Meal planning, experimenting with new foods, and forming enduring habits are some examples of how to achieve this.

3.3 Incorporating Low-Sodium and High-Potassium Foods

1. Prioritize Low-Sodium Options:

- **Read Labels:** When shopping, read the nutrition labels. Select packaged meals, condiments, and canned items that have low or no added salt.
- **Fresh is Best:** Pick entire foods and fresh produce over processed ones whenever you can. Naturally, fresh foods have reduced salt content.

2. Enhance Flavor Naturally:

- **Herbs and Spices:** Instead of using salt to flavor your food, use a range of herbs and spices. Try different mixes to get intriguing new flavor characteristics.
- **Citrus Juices:** Add zest to your food by using citrus juices like lime or lemon. These enhance the flavor of your food while also adding to its total nutritious value.

3. Embrace High-Potassium Foods:

- **Bananas:** Add fruits high in potassium, such as bananas, to your meals and snacks.
- **Leafy Greens:** As a great source of potassium, choose leafy green veggies like kale and spinach.

- **Beans and Lentils:** To increase your intake of potassium, include a range of beans and lentils in your meals.
- **Potassium-Rich Proteins:** Select lean meats, fish, and chicken as examples of proteins high in potassium.

4. Plan Balanced Meals:

- **Consider the Ratio:** Aim for mealtime potassium to sodium ratio that is in equilibrium. This helps control blood pressure and maintains general electrolyte balance.
- **Diverse Protein Sources:** To guarantee a complete nutrient profile, incorporate a variety of protein sources into your meals. This can apply to both plant- and animal-based diets.

5. Hydration Matters:

- **Water Consumption:** Drink lots of water to be well hydrated. Hydration is important for maintaining electrolyte balance and overall health.

6. Limit Processed and Fast Foods:

- **Hidden Sodium:** Fast food and processed foods are common sources of unrecognized salt. Restricting these foods helps you follow the DASH Diet's guidelines and lowers your overall salt intake.

You can create a heart-healthy and long-lasting dietary plan by thoroughly comprehending the DASH Diet principles, modifying the diet to fit your needs, and including foods high in potassium and low in salt. We'll be turning these ideas into doable, tasty, and effortlessly made foods in the upcoming chapters as we go with "The DASH DIET MEAL PREP." Prepare to taste the flavors of vigor and health!

Chapter 4: Weekly Meal Plans

This chapter of "The DASH DIET MEAL PREP: Delectable Recipes for Heart Health" In "Low-Sodium, High-Potassium to Control Blood Pressure," we'll focus on meal planning's usefulness. This chapter contains meal plans for all skill levels, from those just beginning to adopt the DASH Diet to those seeking more complex meal plans for sustained success. We'll also talk about how to add variety and make sure you're getting a balanced supply of vital nutrients.

4.1 Sample Meal Plans for Beginners

Starting a new diet regimen may be thrilling as well as difficult. It's crucial to begin with easy, tasty, and doable meal ideas if you're a newbie. Here are some days' worth of sample meal plans to get you started on the DASH Diet:

Day 1:

Breakfast:

- Greek Yogurt Parfait with Fresh Berries and a Drizzle of Honey

- Whole Grain Toast with Avocado Slices

Lunch:

- Quinoa Salad with Cherry Tomatoes, Cucumbers, and Feta Cheese
- Grilled Chicken Breast

Dinner:

- Baked Salmon with Lemon-Dill Sauce
- Steamed Broccoli
- Brown Rice

Snack:

- Apple Slices with Almond Butter

Day 2:

Breakfast:

- Spinach and Feta Omelette
- Whole Wheat English Muffin

Lunch:

- Lentil and Vegetable Soup
- Mixed Green Salad with Olive Oil and Lemon Dressing

Dinner:

- Turkey and Vegetable Stir-Fry
- Quinoa

Snack:

- Carrot Sticks with Hummus

Day 3:

Breakfast:

- Berry Smoothie Bowl with Greek Yogurt and Granola
- Whole Grain Banana Muffin

Lunch:

- Chickpea Salad with Tomatoes, Cucumbers, and Red Onion
- Grilled Shrimp Skewers

Dinner:

- Vegetable and Bean Burrito Bowl with Brown Rice
- Guacamole and Salsa

Snack:

- Mixed Nuts and Dried Fruits

These sample meal plans provide an overview of the delectable and varied options that fall within the framework of the DASH Diet. When starting off, concentrate on including a range of nutritious grains, fruits, vegetables, lean meats, and healthy fats in your meals. Try a variety of recipes to find one that works well for your schedule and your taste preferences.

4.2 Advanced Meal Plans for Long-Term Success

After you've mastered the fundamentals of the DASH Diet, you can go on to more complicated meal plans that offer more diversity and nutritional complexity. For a day planned with long-term success in mind, consider these sample meal plans:

Day 1:

Breakfast:

- Spinach and Mushroom Frittata with Whole Grain Toast
- Fresh Fruit Salad

Lunch:

- Quinoa and Black Bean Stuffed Bell Peppers
- Greek Salad with Olives and Feta

Dinner:

- Grilled Halibut with Mango Salsa
- Roasted Sweet Potato Wedges
- Quinoa Pilaf with Mixed Vegetables

Snack:

- Greek Yogurt with Chia Seeds and Berries

Day 2:

Breakfast:

- Overnight Oats with Almond Milk, Chia Seeds, and Mixed Berries
- Whole Grain Banana Bread

Lunch:

- Lentil and Kale Soup
- Avocado and Chickpea Wrap with Whole Wheat Tortilla

Dinner:

- Baked Chicken Thighs with Rosemary and Lemon
- Steamed Asparagus with Lemon Zest
- Wild Rice Blend

Snack:

- Edamame and Cherry Tomato Skewers

Day 3:

Breakfast:

- Acai Bowl with Granola, Coconut, and Fresh Fruit
- Whole Wheat Blueberry Muffins

Lunch:

- Salmon and Avocado Salad with Quinoa and Lemon-Dijon Dressing
- Whole Grain Crackers

Dinner:

- Stir-Fried Tofu with Broccoli and Snow Peas
- Brown Rice Noodles with Sesame-Ginger Sauce

Snack:

Cottage Cheese with Pineapple Chunks

With a greater variety of products and cooking methods, these advanced meal plans offer a sophisticated gastronomic experience while still following the DASH Diet's guidelines. Feel free to experiment with more recipes as you go along and modify meal plans to fit your changing dietary needs.

4.3 Tips for Variety and Nutrient Balance

Sustaining a good DASH Diet requires keeping things varied and obtaining a balance of vital nutrients. The following advice can help to maximize diversity and nutrient intake:

1. Explore Different Cuisines:

- **International Flavors:** Try out different dishes to introduce new ingredients and flavors. Latin American, Asian, and Mediterranean cuisines frequently provide heart-healthy choices that complement the DASH Diet.

2. Local and Seasonal Produce:

- **Incorporate Seasonality:** Use Seasonality Accept seasonal vegetables to maintain the freshness and variety of your meals all year long. Go to your neighborhood farmers' markets to find unusual and regional foods.

3. Rotate Protein Sources:

- **Diverse Proteins:** Include a mix of animal and plant-based proteins in your meals. Rotate between poultry, fish, lean meats, beans, lentils, and tofu to ensure a diverse range of amino acids and nutrients.

4. Colorful Plate:

- **Variety of Colors:** Use a wide variety of fruits and vegetables to create a colorful plate. Variations in color frequently correspond to different nutrient profiles, offering a broad range of vitamins and minerals.

5. Whole Grains and Fiber:

- **Explore Whole Grains:** To give your dishes more texture and nutritional diversity, try different whole grains like barley, quinoa, and farro. To enhance digestive health, prioritize high-fiber foods.

6. Healthy Fats:

- **Omega-3 Rich Foods:** To support heart health, eat foods high in omega-3s, such as walnuts, flaxseeds, and fatty fish. These beneficial fats support general health.

7. Mindful Eating:

- **Savor the Flavors:** In order to practice mindful eating, take time to appreciate each mouthful of your food and pay attention to its flavors and textures. In addition to improving the eating experience, this promotes a positive relationship with food.

8. Nutritional Tracking:

- **Monitor Nutrient Intake:** To keep track of the nutrients you consume each day, try utilizing a journal or an app for nutrition tracking. This can make sure you reach your dietary objectives and point out areas that need improvement.

9. Hydration:

- **Water and Herbal Teas:** Stay well-hydrated by drinking plenty of water throughout the day. Consider incorporating herbal teas for additional flavor without added calories or sugar.

10. Adapt and Evolve:

- **Personalize Your Diet:** Over time, your nutritional requirements and preferences could change. To keep your diet pleasurable and sustainable, be willing to make adjustments to your meal plans as needed.

As you put these suggestions into practice, keep in mind that diversity and nutrient balance are important for your general health and wellbeing as well as for the DASH Diet's success.

Take advantage of the chance to experiment with different foods, flavors, and cooking techniques to ensure that your experience with "The DASH DIET MEAL PREP" is rewarding and pleasurable. We will expand on these ideas in the next chapters and provide you a wide variety of mouthwatering, heart-healthy dishes. Prepare to improve your cooking abilities and fuel your body with the finest foods the DASH Diet has to offer!

Chapter 5: Heart-Healthy Breakfast Recipes

Greetings from breakfast, the center of your day! Here in this chapter of "The DASH DIET MEAL PREP: Delicious Heart-Healthy Recipes Low-Sodium, High-Potassium to Manage Blood Pressure," we'll look at hearty breakfast options that will not only get you going in the morning but also support the DASH Diet rules. Prepare to enjoy the tasty goodness of unique avocado toast variations, whole grain breakfast muffins, and revitalizing smoothie bowls.

5.1 Energizing Smoothie Bowls

Smoothie bowls are a tasty and wholesome way to start the day. Tightly packed with a variety of fruits, veggies, and other healthful components, they provide a taste explosion along with vital nutrients. Here are two recipes for energetic smoothie bowls that will make breakfast more enjoyable:

Recipe 1: Berry Blast Smoothie Bowl

Ingredients:

- 1 cup mixed berries (strawberries, blueberries, raspberries)
- 1 ripe banana, frozen
- 1/2 cup Greek yogurt
- 1/4 cup almond milk
- 1 tablespoon chia seeds
- Toppings: sliced strawberries, granola, and a drizzle of honey

Instructions:

1. In a blender, combine the mixed berries, frozen banana, Greek yogurt, and almond milk.
2. Blend until smooth and creamy, adding more almond milk if needed to reach your desired consistency.
3. Pour the smoothie into a bowl.
4. Top with sliced strawberries, granola, and a drizzle of honey.
5. Enjoy with a spoon, savoring the vibrant flavors and textures.

Recipe 2: Green Goddess Smoothie Bowl

Ingredients:

- 1 cup spinach leaves
- 1/2 avocado
- 1/2 cucumber, peeled
- 1/2 green apple, cored
- 1/2 cup coconut water
- 1 tablespoon flaxseeds
- Toppings: kiwi slices, coconut flakes, and pumpkin seeds

Instructions:

1. In a blender, combine the spinach leaves, avocado, cucumber, green apple, and coconut water.
2. Blend until smooth and creamy.
3. Add flaxseeds and blend briefly to incorporate.
4. Pour the green smoothie into a bowl.
5. Top with kiwi slices, coconut flakes, and pumpkin seeds.
6. Dive into this nutrient-packed bowl to fuel your morning with green goodness.

Smoothie bowls offer a great way to tailor your breakfast to your personal preferences. To keep your breakfast routine interesting and fulfilling, try experimenting with different fruit combinations, additions, and toppings.

5.2 Whole Grain Breakfast Muffins

For hectic mornings, muffins make a handy and portable breakfast alternative that can be made ahead of time. Breakfast can be made tasty and heart-healthy by adding nuts, fruits, and whole grains. Two recipes for whole grain breakfast muffins are provided below:

Recipe 1: Blueberry Oat Muffins

Ingredients:

- 1 cup rolled oats
- 1 cup whole wheat flour
- 1/2 cup almond flour
- 1 teaspoon baking powder
- 1/2 teaspoon baking soda
- 1/4 teaspoon salt
- 1/2 cup Greek yogurt
- 1/4 cup honey
- 2 ripe bananas, mashed
- 2 large eggs
- 1 teaspoon vanilla extract

- 1 cup blueberries (fresh or frozen)
- Topping: sliced almonds

Instructions:

1. Preheat the oven to 350°F (175°C) and line a muffin tin with paper liners.
2. In a large bowl, combine rolled oats, whole wheat flour, almond flour, baking powder, baking soda, and salt.
3. In a separate bowl, whisk together Greek yogurt, honey, mashed bananas, eggs, and vanilla extract.
4. Add the wet ingredients to the dry ingredients and mix until just combined.
5. Gently fold in the blueberries.
6. Divide the batter evenly among the muffin cups and sprinkle sliced almonds on top.
7. Bake for 18-20 minutes or until a toothpick inserted into the center comes out clean.
8. Allow the muffins to cool before enjoying these wholesome and flavorful treats.

Recipe 2: Apple Cinnamon Quinoa Muffins

Ingredients:

- 1 cup cooked quinoa, cooled
- 1 cup whole wheat flour

- 1/2 cup almond flour
- 1 teaspoon baking powder
- 1/2 teaspoon baking soda
- 1/2 teaspoon ground cinnamon
- 1/4 teaspoon salt
- 1/2 cup unsweetened applesauce
- 1/4 cup maple syrup
- 2 large eggs
- 1 teaspoon vanilla extract
- 1 apple, finely diced
- Topping: chopped walnuts

Instructions:

1. Preheat the oven to 350°F (175°C) and line a muffin tin with paper liners.
2. In a large bowl, combine cooked quinoa, whole wheat flour, almond flour, baking powder, baking soda, ground cinnamon, and salt.
3. In another bowl, whisk together applesauce, maple syrup, eggs, and vanilla extract.
4. Add the wet ingredients to the dry ingredients and mix until just combined.
5. Fold in the diced apple.
6. Divide the batter among the muffin cups and sprinkle chopped walnuts on top.

7. Bake for 20-22 minutes or until a toothpick inserted into the center comes out clean.

8. Allow the muffins to cool before indulging in these nutritious and satisfying treats.

Make whole grain muffins ahead of time and put them in the fridge for an easy grab-and-go breakfast. To make variants that fit your tastes, feel free to experiment with different fruits, nuts, and spices.

5.3 Avocado Toast Variations

Because of its ease of use and adaptability, avocado toast has become a breakfast classic. You can make this simple dish into a tasty and nutritious breakfast option by adding different toppings to it. To improve your morning meal, try these two variations on avocado toast:

Recipe 1: Mediterranean Avocado Toast

Ingredients:

- 1 slice whole grain bread, toasted
- 1/2 avocado, mashed
- 1 tablespoon hummus

- Cherry tomatoes, halved

- Cucumber slices

- Kalamata olives, sliced

- Feta cheese, crumbled

- Fresh basil leaves

- Olive oil for drizzling

- Salt and pepper to taste

Instructions:

1. Toast the whole grain bread to your liking.

2. Spread the mashed avocado evenly over the toast.

3. Spoon hummus on top of the avocado layer.

4. Arrange halved cherry tomatoes, cucumber slices, and sliced Kalamata olives on the toast.

5. Crumble feta cheese over the vegetables.

6. Garnish with fresh basil leaves.

7. Drizzle olive oil over the toast and season with salt and pepper to taste.

8. Enjoy this Mediterranean-inspired avocado toast for a flavorful and satisfying breakfast.

Recipe 2: Smoked Salmon and Egg Avocado Toast

Ingredients:

- 1 slice whole grain bread, toasted

- 1/2 avocado, sliced

- Smoked salmon

- Poached or fried egg

- Capers

- Red onion, thinly sliced

- Fresh dill

- Lemon wedge

- Salt and pepper to taste

Instructions:

1. Toast the whole grain bread to your liking.

2. Arrange sliced avocado on top of the toast.

3. Drape smoked salmon over the avocado.

4. Place a poached or fried egg on top of the salmon.

5. Scatter capers and thinly sliced red onion over the toast.

6. Garnish with fresh dill.

7. Squeeze a lemon wedge over the toast for a burst of citrus flavor.

8. Sprinkle with salt and pepper to taste.

9. Delight in this elegant and protein-rich avocado toast for a sophisticated breakfast experience.

Various avocado toast options let you express your creativity and customize your meal to fit your dietary requirements and mood. To keep your breakfast routine interesting and nourishing, experiment with different toppings, textures, and taste profiles.

Remember to appreciate the nourishment your body is receiving with every bite as you add these heart-healthy breakfast foods into your DASH Diet meal plan. We'll continue our culinary adventure with more delectable lunch, dinner, and snack recipes in the upcoming chapters, guaranteeing a varied and fulfilling experience with "The DASH DIET MEAL PREP." Prepare to taste new tastes, improve your cooking abilities, and follow the road to better health!

Chapter 6: Nutrient-Packed Lunch Ideas

Lunch is a great time to give your body a nutritional boost with foods that follow the DASH Diet's guidelines. This chapter of "The DASH DIET MEAL PREP: Delectable Recipes for Heart Health" Using the theme "Low-Sodium, High-Potassium to Manage Blood Pressure," we'll look at energizing lunch ideas that combine a range of tastes and textures. Prepare to savor quinoa power bowls, vibrant salad jars, and mouthwatering grilled chicken wraps that will satisfy your palate as well as your body.

6.1 Colorful Salad Jars

A tasty and eye-catching way to eat a nutrient-rich lunch is using salad jars. You may make a dinner that is both portable and customized, and that keeps fresh until you're ready to eat it, by layering colorful ingredients in a jar. Here are two recipes to liven up your noon snack: vibrant salad jars

Recipe 1: Mediterranean Chickpea Salad Jar

Ingredients:

- 1/4 cup balsamic vinaigrette dressing
- 1/2 cup cherry tomatoes, halved
- 1/2 cucumber, diced
- 1/4 cup Kalamata olives, sliced
- 1/4 cup red onion, finely chopped
- 1/2 cup chickpeas, cooked
- 1 cup mixed greens (spinach, arugula, or your choice)
- Feta cheese, crumbled (optional)
- Fresh basil leaves for garnish

Assembly:

1. Start by adding balsamic vinaigrette dressing to the bottom of a mason jar.
2. Layer cherry tomatoes, cucumber, Kalamata olives, red onion, and chickpeas in the jar.
3. Add mixed greens on top, pressing them down gently to fit more.
4. If using, sprinkle crumbled feta cheese on the greens.
5. Seal the jar and refrigerate until ready to eat.
6. When ready to enjoy, shake the jar to distribute the dressing, and pour the contents into a bowl.

7. Garnish with fresh basil leaves and relish the Mediterranean flavors.

Recipe 2: Rainbow Quinoa Salad Jar

Ingredients:

- 1/4 cup lemon-tahini dressing
- 1/2 cup cooked quinoa, cooled
- 1/2 cup red bell pepper, diced
- 1/2 cup carrot, shredded
- 1/2 cup yellow bell pepper, diced
- 1/2 cup edamame, shelled
- 1/2 cup purple cabbage, thinly sliced
- 1 cup kale, finely chopped
- Pumpkin seeds for garnish

Assembly:

1. Begin by pouring lemon-tahini dressing into the bottom of a mason jar.
2. Add a layer of cooked quinoa, followed by diced red bell pepper, shredded carrot, diced yellow bell pepper, edamame, sliced purple cabbage, and chopped kale.
3. Top with pumpkin seeds for added crunch.
4. Seal the jar and refrigerate until lunchtime.

5. When ready to eat, shake the jar to evenly distribute the dressing, and transfer the contents into a bowl.

6. Enjoy a vibrant and nutrient-packed rainbow quinoa salad.

Try a variety of dressings, veggies, and protein sources to customize salad jars to your liking. To keep ingredients fresh and avoid sogginess, layering them judiciously is crucial.

6.2 Quinoa Power Bowls

Quinoa power bowls are a flexible and high-protein lunch choice that let you put together a range of toppings for a filling meal. Because of their adaptability, you can easily customize these bowls to fit your dietary requirements and taste preferences. To improve your lunchtime experience, try these two recipes for quinoa power bowls:

Recipe 1: Southwest Quinoa Power Bowl

Ingredients:

- 1 cup cooked quinoa, cooled
- 1/2 cup black beans, canned and rinsed
- 1/2 cup corn kernels, cooked
- 1/2 cup cherry tomatoes, halved

- 1/4 cup red onion, finely chopped
- 1/2 avocado, sliced
- 1/4 cup cilantro, chopped
- Lime wedges for serving

Instructions:

1. In a bowl, assemble the cooked quinoa as the base.
2. Arrange black beans, corn kernels, cherry tomatoes, red onion, and sliced avocado on top.
3. Sprinkle chopped cilantro over the bowl.
4. Serve with lime wedges on the side for a burst of citrus flavor.
5. Toss the ingredients together before eating; ensuring every bite is a delightful blend of Southwest-inspired goodness.

Recipe 2: Mediterranean Quinoa Power Bowl

Ingredients:

- 1 cup cooked quinoa, cooled
- 1/2 cup hummus
- 1/2 cup cucumber, diced
- 1/2 cup cherry tomatoes, halved
- 1/4 cup Kalamata olives, sliced
- 1/4 cup red onion, finely chopped
- Feta cheese, crumbled

- Fresh parsley for garnish

Instructions:

1. Begin by spreading a layer of hummus at the bottom of a bowl.
2. Add the cooked quinoa as the next layer.
3. Arrange diced cucumber, cherry tomatoes, sliced Kalamata olives, and finely chopped red onion on top.
4. Sprinkle crumbled feta cheese over the bowl.
5. Garnish with fresh parsley for a burst of herbaceous flavor.
6. Mix the ingredients together before indulging in this Mediterranean-inspired quinoa power bowl.

Quinoa power bowls deliver a healthy dose of nutrients along with a tasty blend of textures and flavors. You can experiment with different proteins, veggies, and dressings to suit your taste when assembling your bowls.

6.3 Grilled Chicken Wraps

Lean protein, a variety of veggies, and tasty sauces are all combined in delicious and portable grilled chicken wraps for lunch. These wraps are a great option for hectic days because they are simple to prepare ahead of time. Here are two recipes for grilled chicken wraps to give your noon meal a savory twist:

Recipe 1: Greek Chicken Wrap

Ingredients:

- 1 boneless, skinless chicken breast, grilled and sliced
- Whole wheat wrap
- Tzatziki sauce
- Cherry tomatoes, halved
- Cucumber, thinly sliced
- Red onion, thinly sliced
- Feta cheese, crumbled
- Fresh oregano leaves for garnish

Instructions:

1. Lay a whole wheat wrap on a clean surface.
2. Spread a generous layer of tzatziki sauce over the wrap.
3. Place grilled and sliced chicken breast on one side of the wrap.
4. Add halved cherry tomatoes, thinly sliced cucumber, and thinly sliced red onion.
5. Sprinkle crumbled feta cheese over the vegetables.
6. Garnish with fresh oregano leaves.

7. Fold the sides of the wrap and roll it tightly.

8. Slice the wrap in half at a diagonal and secure with toothpicks if needed.

9. Enjoy this Greek-inspired grilled chicken wrap that bursts with Mediterranean flavors.

Recipe 2: BBQ Chicken and Avocado Wrap

Ingredients:

- 1 boneless, skinless chicken breast, grilled and sliced
- Whole wheat wrap
- BBQ sauce
- Avocado, sliced
- Red cabbage, shredded
- Fresh cilantro leaves
- Lime wedges for serving

Instructions:

1. Place a whole wheat wrap on a clean surface.
2. Drizzle a layer of BBQ sauce over the wrap.
3. Arrange grilled and sliced chicken breast on one side of the wrap.
4. Add sliced avocado, shredded red cabbage, and fresh cilantro leaves.
5. Squeeze lime wedges over the ingredients for a zesty kick.

6. Fold the sides of the wrap and roll it tightly.

7. Slice the wrap in half at a diagonal for easy handling.

8. Indulge in the delicious combination of BBQ chicken and creamy avocado in every bite.

Lunchtime grilled chicken wraps are a filling and tasty choice because they offer a good ratio of protein, fiber, and healthy fats. For an added personal touch, add your preferred sauces, extra toppings, and veggies to the wraps.

As you incorporate these nutrient-dense lunch ideas into your meal planning for the DASH Diet, keep in mind that keeping your eating habits interesting and healthy requires diversity. We will continue to delve into delectable dinner, snack, and dessert recipes in the next chapters, guaranteeing a varied and rewarding culinary experience with "The DASH DIET MEAL PREP." Prepare to enhance your food, fuel your body, and welcome the path to greater health!

Chapter 7: Nourishing Dinner Options

Dinner is a vital component of your day since it provides you with a chance to relax and refuel with heart-healthy, nutritious food. This chapter of "The DASH DIET MEAL PREP: Delectable Recipes for Heart Health" In "Low-Sodium, High-Potassium to Control Blood Pressure," we'll look at filling dinner choices that follow the DASH Diet's guidelines. Get ready to enjoy the delights of turkey and vegetable stuffed peppers, a vegetable stir-fry with tofu, and baked fish with lemon-dill sauce.

7.1 Baked Salmon with Lemon-Dill Sauce

In addition to being delicious and high in nutrients, salmon is a great source of omega-3 fatty acids, which are known to promote heart health. Salmon gets a flavor boost from baking it with a tart lemon-dill sauce, which also keeps the meal light and crisp. To make this delicious supper choice, follow these steps:

Ingredients:

- 4 salmon fillets
- 1 tablespoon olive oil

- Salt and pepper to taste
- 2 tablespoons fresh dill, chopped
- 1 lemon, sliced
- Lemon-Dill Sauce:
- 1/4 cup plain Greek yogurt
- 1 tablespoon Dijon mustard
- 1 tablespoon fresh lemon juice
- 1 tablespoon fresh dill, chopped
- Salt and pepper to taste

Instructions:

1. Preheat the oven to 400°F (200°C) and line a baking sheet with parchment paper.
2. Place the salmon fillets on the prepared baking sheet.
3. Drizzle olive oil over the salmon and season with salt and pepper.
4. Sprinkle chopped fresh dill over the fillets.
5. Arrange lemon slices on top of the salmon.
6. Bake in the preheated oven for 12-15 minutes or until the salmon flakes easily with a fork.
7. While the salmon is baking, prepare the lemon-dill sauce by whisking together Greek yogurt, Dijon mustard, lemon juice, chopped dill, salt, and pepper in a bowl.
8. Once the salmon is done, serve each fillet with a dollop of lemon-dill sauce on top.

9. Garnish with additional fresh dill and lemon wedges if desired.

10. Enjoy a nourishing dinner that's not only heart-healthy but also bursting with delightful flavors.

7.2 Vegetable Stir-Fry with Tofu

Stir-fries are great ways to add a range of vibrant veggies to your dinner, making it a filling and nutrient-rich dish. By including tofu, you can add plant-based protein to this recipe, giving it a well-rounded option for people looking for a vegan, heart-healthy option. Here's how to make a tasty tofu-based vegetable stir-fry:

Ingredients:

- 14 oz (400g) extra-firm tofu, pressed and cubed
- 2 tablespoons soy sauce (low-sodium)
- 1 tablespoon sesame oil
- 1 tablespoon corn-starch
- 1 tablespoon vegetable oil
- 3 cups mixed vegetables (broccoli, bell peppers, carrots, snap peas)
- 3 cloves garlic, minced
- 1 tablespoon fresh ginger, grated
- Cooked brown rice for serving

- Sesame seeds and green onions for garnish

Instructions:

1. In a bowl, combine cubed tofu with soy sauce, sesame oil, and corn-starch. Toss to coat the tofu evenly.
2. Heat vegetable oil in a large wok or skillet over medium-high heat.
3. Add marinated tofu to the pan and cook until golden brown on all sides. Remove tofu from the pan and set aside.
4. In the same pan, add a bit more oil if needed, and sauté garlic and ginger until fragrant.
5. Add mixed vegetables to the pan and stir-fry until they are tender-crisp.
6. Return the cooked tofu to the pan and toss everything together until well combined.
7. Serve the vegetable stir-fry over cooked brown rice.
8. Garnish with sesame seeds and chopped green onions.
9. Enjoy a vibrant and nutrient-packed dinner that's not only delicious but also supports your heart health.

7.3 Turkey and Vegetable Stuffed Peppers

A tasty and inventive way to include lean protein and a range of veggies in your dinner is with stuffed peppers. This dish is tasty and substantial, made with ground turkey, nutritious grains, and a colorful variety of vegetables. Here's how to make veggie-stuffed peppers and turkey:

Ingredients:

- 4 large bell peppers, halved and seeds removed
- 1 tablespoon olive oil
- 1 pound (450g) lean ground turkey
- 1 onion, finely chopped
- 2 cloves garlic, minced
- 1 zucchini, diced
- 1 cup cooked quinoa
- 1 cup cherry tomatoes, halved
- 1 teaspoon dried oregano
- 1 teaspoon ground cumin
- Salt and pepper to taste
- 1 cup tomato sauce
- 1/2 cup low-sodium chicken broth
- 1/2 cup shredded mozzarella cheese
- Fresh parsley for garnish

Instructions:

1. Preheat the oven to 375°F (190°C).
2. Heat olive oil in a large skillet over medium heat.

3. Add ground turkey and cook until browned, breaking it apart with a spoon as it cooks.

4. Add chopped onion and minced garlic to the skillet, sautéing until the onion is translucent.

5. Stir in diced zucchini, cooked quinoa, cherry tomatoes, dried oregano, ground cumin, salt, and pepper. Cook for an additional 2-3 minutes.

6. In a separate bowl, mix tomato sauce and chicken broth.

7. Pour a small amount of the tomato sauce mixture into the bottom of a baking dish.

8. Arrange halved bell peppers in the baking dish.

9. Stuff each pepper half with the turkey and vegetable mixture.

10. Pour the remaining tomato sauce mixture over the stuffed peppers.

11. Cover the baking dish with aluminum foil and bake in the preheated oven for 25-30 minutes, or until the peppers are tender.

12. Remove the foil, sprinkle shredded mozzarella cheese over the stuffed peppers, and bake for an additional 5 minutes, or until the cheese is melted and bubbly.

13. Garnish with fresh parsley before serving.

14. Delight in these turkey and vegetable stuffed peppers for a hearty and nutritious dinner.

These heart-healthy supper ideas not only add taste and diversity to your evening meals, but they also improve heart health. As you go with "The DASH DIET MEAL PREP," keep in mind that general wellbeing is influenced by a varied and well-balanced diet. We'll go over delicious recipes for appetizers, sweets, and more in the next chapters, so your culinary journey stays fulfilling and health-conscious. Prepare to appreciate the advantages of the DASH Diet and learn more delectable methods to fuel your body!

Chapter 8: Snacks and Sides for Every Occasion

When it comes to heart-healthy eating, snacks and sides are essential for sustaining energy levels and warding off hunger. In "The DASH DIET MEAL PREP: Delicious Heart-Healthy Recipes Low-Sodium, High-Potassium to Manage Blood Pressure," this chapter will cover tasty options that satisfy and nourish at various times. Prepare to savor the delightfully creamy guacamole with vegetable sticks, the crispy sweetness of roasted chickpeas, and the cool layers of a Greek yogurt parfait.

8.1 Roasted Chickpeas

Roasted chickpeas are a crisp and adaptable snack that can be a great substitute for traditional less healthful alternatives. Chickpeas offer a nutrient-dense basis that can be tailored with different spices to suit your taste preferences. They are high in protein and fiber. This is how to make this tasty snack:

Ingredients:

- 2 cans (15 oz each) chickpeas, drained and rinsed
- 2 tablespoons olive oil

- 1 teaspoon ground cumin

- 1 teaspoon smoked paprika

- 1/2 teaspoon garlic powder

- 1/2 teaspoon onion powder

- 1/4 teaspoon cayenne pepper (optional)

- Salt and black pepper to taste

Instructions:

1. Preheat the oven to 400°F (200°C) and line a baking sheet with parchment paper.

2. Rinse and thoroughly dry the chickpeas using a clean kitchen towel or paper towels.

3. In a bowl, toss the chickpeas with olive oil, ground cumin, smoked paprika, garlic powder, onion powder, cayenne pepper (if using), salt, and black pepper.

4. Spread the seasoned chickpeas evenly on the prepared baking sheet.

5. Roast in the preheated oven for 25-30 minutes, or until the chickpeas are golden brown and crispy.

6. Shake the baking sheet or stir the chickpeas every 10 minutes to ensure even roasting.

7. Once done, remove from the oven and let the roasted chickpeas cool before enjoying.

8. Store in an airtight container for up to a week.

In addition to being a tasty snack on their own, roasted chickpeas can be added in a variety of ways to salads, soups, and trail mixes. Try blending several spices to make unique combinations that will pique your interest.

8.2 Guacamole with Veggie Sticks

The freshness of tomatoes, onions, and limes combine with the creamy richness of avocados to create a heart-healthy dip known as guacamole. When paired with vibrant vegetable sticks, it transforms into a tasty and nutrient-dense snack or side dish. Here's how to make an easy yet delectable guacamole:

Guacamole Ingredients:

- 3 ripe avocados, peeled and pitted
- 1 small red onion, finely diced
- 2 tomatoes, diced
- 1-2 cloves garlic, minced
- 1 lime, juiced
- 1/4 cup fresh cilantro, chopped
- Salt and pepper to taste
- Veggie Sticks:
- Carrot sticks
- Cucumber slices

- Bell pepper strips (assorted colors)
- Celery sticks

Instructions:

1. In a bowl, mash the ripe avocados with a fork.
2. Add diced red onion, diced tomatoes, minced garlic, lime juice, and chopped cilantro to the mashed avocados.
3. Season with salt and pepper to taste.
4. Mix all the ingredients until well combined.
5. Adjust lime, salt, and pepper according to your taste preferences.
6. Cover the guacamole with plastic wrap, ensuring it touches the surface to prevent browning.
7. Refrigerate for at least 30 minutes before serving to allow the flavors to meld.
8. Serve the guacamole with an assortment of veggie sticks for a refreshing and nutrient-packed snack.

Not only is guacamole a tasty dip, but it can also be used as a variety of toppings for fish, grilled chicken, or whole grain bread. To add more taste variety, feel free to get creative and add additional ingredients like sliced mango or jalapeños.

8.3 Greek Yogurt Parfait

The delicious blend of creamy yogurt, crunchy toppings, and fresh fruits is found in Greek yogurt parfaits. This adaptable delicacy can be had as a light breakfast, as a nutritious dessert, or as a snack. This is how to put together a Greek yogurt parfait that is heart-healthy:

Ingredients:

- 2 cups plain Greek yogurt
- 1 cup mixed berries (strawberries, blueberries, raspberries)
- 1/4 cup granola (low-sugar)
- 2 tablespoons honey or maple syrup
- 1/4 cup chopped nuts (almonds, walnuts, or pistachios)
- Fresh mint leaves for garnish

Instructions:

1. In a glass or a bowl, start by layering a portion of plain Greek yogurt.
2. Add a layer of mixed berries on top of the yogurt.
3. Sprinkle a portion of granola over the berries.
4. Drizzle honey or maple syrup over the granola layer.
5. Repeat the layers until you fill the glass or bowl.
6. Finish with a sprinkle of chopped nuts.

7. Garnish with fresh mint leaves for a burst of freshness.

8. Serve immediately and enjoy the delicious combination of textures and flavors.

Parfaits made with Greek yogurt are quite customisable; you may play around with different types of fruit, nuts, and toppings. This adaptable confection offers a gratifying combination of fiber, protein, and natural sweetness without having too many added sweets.

While you peruse these appetizers and accompaniments, keep in mind that maintaining a heart-healthy lifestyle requires balance and moderation. These choices not only boost your daily intake of nutrients, but they also liven up your meals and snacks. We'll continue our culinary exploration in the next chapters with delicious dessert ideas and advice on how to stick to a fun and sustainable DASH Diet. As you set out on your journey to improved heart health, get ready to uncover even more delectable dishes and insights!

Chapter 9: Desserts That Satisfy Sweet Cravings

You don't have to give up on your sweet craving when following the DASH Diet to start your journey toward heart health. This chapter of "The DASH DIET MEAL PREP: Delectable Recipes for Heart Health" Low-Sodium, High-Potassium Blood Pressure Management," we'll look at delicious treats that put flavor first without sacrificing your heart health commitment. Prepare to savor the wholesome charm of banana-oat biscuits, the rich and nutty taste of dark chocolate and nut clusters, and the refreshing sweetness of berry medley popsicles.

9.1 Berry Medley Popsicles

Especially in the warmer months, popsicles are a cold and refreshing treat that you can make at home with full control over the sugar and ingredient content. The natural sweetness of berries and the moisturizing properties of coconut water are combined in these berry medley popsicles. Here's how to make this easy dessert that tastes delicious:

Ingredients:

- 1 cup mixed berries (strawberries, blueberries, raspberries)
- 2 cups coconut water
- 1-2 tablespoons honey or maple syrup (optional, depending on sweetness preference)
- 1 teaspoon vanilla extract (optional)

Instructions:

1. Rinse the mixed berries and slice larger berries, if needed.
2. In a blender, combine the mixed berries, coconut water, honey or maple syrup (if using), and vanilla extract (if using).
3. Blend until smooth.
4. Taste the mixture and adjust sweetness, if necessary.
5. Pour the berry mixture into Popsicle molds.
6. Insert Popsicle sticks into the molds.
7. Freeze for at least 4-6 hours or until fully set.
8. Once frozen, run the molds under warm water to release the popsicles.
9. Enjoy these berry medley popsicles for a guilt-free and refreshing dessert.

Try varying the berry combinations you use, or for a zesty touch, squeeze in some fresh lemon juice. These popsicles provide you a boost of antioxidants and water in addition to satisfying your sweet tooth.

9.2 Dark Chocolate and Nut Clusters

Because of its antioxidant qualities, dark chocolate can be included in a diet that promotes heart health when eaten in moderation. This dessert transforms into a filling and healthy treat when paired with nuts, which are high in heart-healthy fats. Here's how to create nut and dark chocolate clusters:

Ingredients:

- 8 oz dark chocolate (70% cocoa or higher), chopped
- 1 cup mixed nuts (almonds, walnuts, pistachios), chopped
- Sea salt for sprinkling (optional)

Instructions:

1. Line a baking sheet with parchment paper.
2. In a heatproof bowl, melt the dark chocolate using a double boiler or in the microwave, stirring every 30 seconds until smooth.
3. Stir in the chopped mixed nuts until they are evenly coated with chocolate.

4. Spoon small clusters of the mixture onto the prepared baking sheet.

5. Sprinkle a pinch of sea salt on top of each cluster, if desired.

6. Place the baking sheet in the refrigerator and chill until the chocolate is set, typically 1-2 hours.

7. Once set, transfer the clusters to an airtight container and store in the refrigerator.

8. Indulge in these dark chocolate and nut clusters when you're in the mood for a rich and satisfying dessert.

These clusters offer a pleasing crunch and a variety of textures in addition to being a lovely sweet treat. Dark chocolate and almonds together create a flavor profile that's heart-healthy and luscious.

9.3 Banana-Oat Cookies

A healthy, naturally sweet dessert alternative with few ingredients is banana-oat cookies. You can alter these gluten-free cookies by adding extra ingredients like dark chocolate chips or almonds. Here's how to whip up these wholesome and simple cookies:

Ingredients:

- 2 ripe bananas, mashed
- 1 cup rolled oats
- 1/4 cup nut butter (almond butter, peanut butter, or your choice)
- 1/4 cup chopped nuts or dark chocolate chips (optional)
- 1/2 teaspoon vanilla extract
- A pinch of cinnamon (optional)

Instructions:

1. Preheat the oven to 350°F (175°C) and line a baking sheet with parchment paper.
2. In a bowl, combine mashed bananas, rolled oats, nut butter, chopped nuts or dark chocolate chips (if using), vanilla extract, and cinnamon (if using).
3. Mix the ingredients until well combined.
4. Drop spoonfuls of the dough onto the prepared baking sheet, shaping them into cookies.
5. Bake in the preheated oven for 12-15 minutes or until the cookies are golden brown.
6. Allow the cookies to cool on the baking sheet for a few minutes before transferring them to a wire rack to cool completely.

7. Enjoy these banana-oat cookies as a guilt-free and wholesome dessert.

You can experiment with different additions, like shredded coconut, dried berries, or chia seeds. Not only are these cookies delicious, but they're also a fantastic way to use up ripe bananas for a gratifying and naturally sweet treat.

When including these treats into your meal planning for the DASH Diet, keep in mind that moderation is essential and that the focus should be on full, nutrient-dense foods. These sweet delights complement your heart-healthy lifestyle by offering a pleasing combination of flavors and textures. We'll conclude our culinary exploration in the last chapter with some extra advice, meal preparation techniques, and a reminder of the delectable options that the DASII Diet offers. Prepare to rejoice in your dedication to heart health and enjoy the benefits of careful and delectable eating!

Chapter 10: DASH Diet Tips for Dining Out

Eating out is a great way to enjoy life while leading a heart-healthy diet. This chapter of "The DASH DIET MEAL PREP: Delectable Recipes for Heart Health" In "Low-Sodium, High-Potassium to Control Blood Pressure," we'll go over helpful advice on how to read restaurant menus, make wise decisions, and adhere to the DASH Diet when dining out. These suggestions will enable you to choose heart-healthy options without sacrificing flavor, whether you're dining out, at a café, or at a social event.

10.1 Making Smart Menu Choices

1. Study the Menu in Advance: If a restaurant has an online menu, spend some time looking it over before you go. This enables you to prepare ahead of time and make wise decisions.

2. Focus on Lean Proteins: Select lean protein foods such grilled chicken, fish, or lentils. Steer clear of highly processed and fried proteins.

3 Load Up on Vegetables: Make a meal that is high in vegetables. Adding additional vegetables to your dinner, whether it's a salad, stir-fry, or entrée made mostly of vegetables, increases its fiber and nutritional value.

4. Be Mindful of Sodium Content: Look out for menu items that can contain a lot of sodium. When it comes to sodium content, "grilled," "steamed," or "roasted" foods tend to be less salty than fried or highly sauced foods.

5. Watch Portion Sizes: Share an entrée or bring leftovers home to reduce wasteful serving sizes. A lot of establishments provide portions larger than what is advised.

6. Choose Whole Grains: Whenever possible, choose whole grains such brown rice, quinoa, or whole wheat pasta. These decisions add to the amount of fiber you consume each day.

7. Ask for Dressings and Sauces on the Side: To help you limit how much you use, ask for dressings and sauces on the side. This enables you to savor the flavors without ingesting an excessive amount of sodium or calories.

8. Skip the Sugary Beverages: Instead of sugary sodas or mixed drinks, go for water, unsweetened tea, or other low-calorie options. Maintaining adequate hydration and limiting additional sugar intake promote heart health.

9. Customize Your Order: Feel free to alter your order to reflect your dietary requirements. A lot of restaurants are open to making adjustments to meet your demands.

10. Balance Your Plate: Make sure your plate has a good mix of whole grains, colorful veggies, lean protein, and healthy fats. This guarantees a filling and varied dinner.

10.2 Requesting Modifications

1. Ask for Grilled or Steamed Options: Rather than having your protein fried, ask to have it grilled or steamed. This lowers the quantity of calories and extra fats in your meal.

2. Substitute Side Dishes: If the typical side dishes don't fit your dietary requirements, request alternatives. For instance, replace fries with steamed veggies or a side salad.

3. Choose Healthy Cooking Oils: Find out what cooking oils are used to prepare meals. Choose to prepare meals with heart-healthy oils such as canola or olive oil.

4. Customize Sauce and Dressing Choices: A lot of foods have dressings or sauces that could be excessively fatty or high in sodium. Ask to have these served on the side, or choose lighter options.

5. Control Cheese and Dairy: Request a smaller quantity or ask for cheese and dairy on the side if a meal has a lot of them. You are now able to regulate how much you eat.

6. Select Whole Grain Options: Ask if you can have a dish with whole grains instead of refined grains, such as white rice or white pasta, if it usually comes with them.

7. Be Clear About Dietary Restrictions: Let your server know if you have any particular dietary requirements or allergies. The majority of places are willing to meet particular dietary requirements.

8. Share Your Preferences Politely: When requesting changes, communicate your preferences in a courteous and understandable manner. Most restaurants will accommodate your dietary requirements as long as they make sense.

9. Request a Box in Advance: When placing an order, request a takeout box if you're worried about the portion sizes. In this manner, you can portion out your meal before you eat.

10. Inquire about Ingredient Substitutes: If a recipe calls for an item that doesn't fit your dietary restrictions, find out what alternatives are available. Alternatives that might better meet your needs can be found at restaurants.

10.3 Staying on Track at Social Gatherings

1. Plan Ahead for Social Events: If you know you'll be attending a social event, make meal plans for the day in advance. To assist prevent extreme hunger; think about having a light, nutrient-dense lunch before the event.

2. Bring a Dish to Share: If the occasion calls for it, serve a dish that promotes heart health with others. This guarantees you a healthy choice and shares delectable, health-conscious recipes with friends and family.

3. Stay Hydrated: To stay hydrated during the event, sip water. This aids in regulating hunger in addition to promoting general wellness.

4. Survey the Food Options: Look over the possibilities for food before adding anything to your plate. Sort the recipes into those that fit the DASH Diet and give them top priority.

5. Practice Mindful Eating: Pay attention to how you eat while you're among other people. Savor the tastes in every bite and be mindful of your body's signals of hunger and fullness.

6. Limit Alcohol Consumption: If alcohol is provided, use it sparingly. Overindulgence in alcohol can result in higher calorie intake and lowered inhibitions, which might cause less conscious eating.

7. Focus on Socializing: Although food is frequently a main attraction at get-togethers, concentrate instead on taking in the companionship of loved ones. Talking to others and doing things together can help de-emphasize eating.

8. Choose Desserts Wisely: If there will be dessert during the event, go for lighter options like fresh fruit or tiny servings of heart-healthy treats. The key is moderation.

9. Be Prepared to Navigate Challenges: Attending social events may bring up unforeseen difficulties, such a lack of healthy options. Remain flexible and take the best decision under the circumstances.

10. Forgive yourself and Move On: If, during a social gathering, you choose unhealthy food, accept responsibility for your actions and move on. Your entire eating pattern is not defined by a single meal or occasion, and each day presents a fresh chance to make heart-healthy decisions.

You can savor the treats of eating out while adhering to the DASH Diet's tenets by using these suggestions for dining out, making adjustments requests, and interacting with social situations. Recall that an approach to eating that is both health-focused and sustainable must include both flexibility and mindfulness. As you wrap up your adventure with "The DASH DIET MEAL PREP," acknowledge the strides you've made and welcome the delectable opportunities that will further enhance your heart-healthy way of living. I toast to your health and the bliss of thoughtful, wholesome eating!

Chapter 11 Maintaining a Healthy Lifestyle beyond the Kitchen

Making dietary and food preparation decisions is only one aspect of starting a heart-healthy journey. In the last chapter of "The DASH DIET MEAL PREP: Delicious Heart-Healthy Recipes Low-Sodium, High-Potassium to Manage Blood Pressure," we'll look at the key elements that go into creating a long-lasting, comprehensive healthy lifestyle. These tactics, which range from tracking your progress and making adjustments to your plan to combining physical activity and stress management techniques, will give you the power to maintain and improve your general well-being.

11.1 Incorporating Physical Activity

A healthy lifestyle is centered on physical activity, which is essential for maintaining cardiovascular health and general wellbeing. Regular exercise is the best way to maximize the benefits of the DASH Diet. The following are methods to make physical activity a part of your everyday schedule:

1. Find Activities You Enjoy: Whether it's swimming, walking, cycling, dancing, or anything else, do something you really enjoy. Exercise becomes a lasting and satisfying component of your routine when it brings you delight.

2. Set Realistic Goals: Make sure your fitness objectives are reasonable and doable. As your fitness level rises, start with short, achievable goals and progressively increase the intensity and time.

3. Create a Consistent Schedule: Arrange your workouts just like you would any other significant appointment. Developing a long-lasting habit requires consistency.

4. Incorporate Cardiovascular and Strength Training: Try to create a well-rounded workout regimen that incorporates both cardiovascular exercises (like jogging or brisk walking) and strength training exercises (like bodyweight exercises and weight lifting). This combo improves general fitness and heart health.

5. Make it Social: Ask loved ones to participate in physical activities with you. Engaging in social activities while exercising, such as a leisure sports league or group exercise, enhances the fun factor.

6. Take Active Breaks: Intersperse brief, vigorous pauses with extended periods of sitting. Throughout the day, take brief walks, stand up, or stretch to rejuvenate your body and mind.

7. Explore Outdoor Activities: Go outside and enjoy things like riding, hiking, and gardening. The benefits of physical activity for overall well-being are amplified when one connects with nature.

8. Use Technology to Stay Motivated: Use wearable, online courses, and fitness applications to monitor your development. Numerous platforms provide a range of exercise programs appropriate for varying degrees of fitness.

9. Prioritize Regular Movement: Adopt a lifestyle that places a premium on movement. When running quick errands, opt to walk or ride your bike instead of using an elevator, and look for ways to fit exercise into your everyday routine.

10. Listen to Your Body: Observe the cues your body is sending you. Speak with a medical expert if you feel pain or discomfort during exercising. Adjust activities as necessary to guarantee fun and safety.

11.2 Stress Management Techniques

A comprehensive approach to well-being must include stress management since long-term stress can have a detrimental effect on heart health. Take into account implementing these stress-reduction strategies into your everyday routine:

1. Practice Mindfulness Meditation: Set aside time for mindfulness meditation every day. To encourage relaxation and mental clarity, pay attention to your breath, your body's sensations, or a guided meditation.

2. Engage in Deep Breathing Exercises: To trigger the body's relaxation response, engage in deep breathing exercises. Breathe in deeply through your nose, hold it for a short while, and then gently release the air through your mouth.

3. Establish a Relaxing Evening Routine: To decompress before going to bed, establish a peaceful evening routine. This could involve doing things like reading, having a warm bath, or doing light stretches.

4. Prioritize Adequate Sleep: Make sure you receive enough good sleep every night. Good sleep supports general health and resilience to stress.

5. Stay Connected with Loved Ones: Make sure you have a close social circle of friends and relatives. Stress is lessened and emotional support is given when experiences, ideas, and feelings are shared with close ones.

6. Engage in Relaxing Hobbies: Make time for enjoyable and stress-relieving activities, such as painting, gardening, or music listening. Stress reduction is achieved by partaking in activities you enjoy.

7. Set Realistic Expectations: Control your expectations and refrain from taking on too much. Prioritize your tasks and set reasonable goals to avoid adding to your stress.

8. Exercise Regularly: Engaging in regular physical activity helps your body and is a great way to decompress. Include enjoyable activities in your schedule on a regular basis.

9. Learn to Delegate: Whether at work or at home, assign duties when you can.

10. Seek Professional Support: Seeking support from a mental health expert is a good idea if stress becomes too much to handle. It can also help to establish a more balanced lifestyle. Counseling or therapy can offer coping mechanisms and techniques for managing stress.

11.3 Tracking Your Progress and Adjusting Your Plan

Monitoring your development is an important way to maintain motivation and make well-informed changes to your lifestyle plan. The following actions can help you keep track of your progress and modify your strategy:

1. Keep a Food and Exercise Journal: Keep a notebook to record your daily dietary intake, physical activity levels, and general state of health. This offers perceptions on trends, achievements, and opportunities for development.

2. Monitor Blood Pressure Regularly: If controlling blood pressure is your main objective, use a home blood pressure monitor to check it on a regular basis. Give your healthcare practitioner this information so they can offer you advice.

3. Set Milestones and Celebrate Achievements: Set attainable goals and acknowledge your progress along the way. Acknowledging accomplishments encourages persistence in effort and reinforces positive behaviors.

4. Adjust Goals as Needed: Evaluate your goals on a regular basis to see if they still fit your priorities and situation. Goals should be modified as necessary to keep them relevant and attainable.

5. Evaluate Dietary Choices: Review your dietary decisions on a regular basis. Are there any areas you might do better? To keep your meals interesting and nourishing, try out different recipes and food combinations.

6. Modify Exercise Routines: To avoid monotony and plateauing, modify your workout regimen. To keep your routine interesting, try adding new exercises, varying the intensity of your workouts, or checking out various fitness classes.

7. Seek Feedback from Professionals: For individualized advice, speak with dietitians, fitness instructors, or medical specialists. Their knowledge can provide insightful advice that is catered to your particular need.

8. Stay Open to Learning: Adopt an attitude of lifelong learning. Keep yourself updated with the most recent findings, dietary recommendations, and workout methods to broaden your understanding and improve your health.

9. Address Setbacks with Compassion: Understand that obstacles are an inevitable part of any trip. Be kind to yourself while approaching them, take what you've learned from it, and utilize it to improve your strategy.

10. Celebrate Your Health Journey: Recognize the effort you've put into improving your health and wellbeing. Honor the beneficial adjustments you've made to your way of life and the effects they've had on your general health.

A sustained and comprehensive approach to health can be achieved by including physical activity, using stress-reduction strategies, and embracing an attitude of continual progress. As you wrap up your adventure with "The DASH DIET MEAL PREP," consider the improvements and behaviors you've established. Never forget that even the smallest action adds up to long-term wellbeing. To a healthy, happy, and heart-filled life!

Chapter 12: Frequently Asked Questions

There are many questions that arise when navigating the DASH Diet and meal preparation. In "The DASH DIET MEAL PREP: Delicious Heart-Healthy Recipes Low-Sodium, High-Potassium to Manage Blood Pressure," we'll go over frequent questions regarding the DASH Diet, offer solutions for meal prep difficulties, and offer advice on getting help from a specialist.

12.1 Common Concerns about the DASH Diet

1. Is the DASH Diet Suitable for Everyone?

- The DASH Diet is generally considered suitable for most adults. However, individuals with specific health conditions or dietary restrictions should consult with a healthcare professional or dietitian before making significant changes to their diet. Pregnant or breastfeeding women may also need modifications to meet their nutritional needs.

2. Can I Follow the DASH Diet if I Have Dietary Restrictions, Such as Gluten Sensitivity?

- Yes, the DASH Diet can be adapted to accommodate various dietary restrictions, including gluten sensitivity. Emphasize naturally gluten-free whole grains like quinoa, brown rice, and oats, and choose gluten-free alternatives for products containing wheat.

3. How Long Does It Take to See Results on the DASH Diet?

- The timeline for seeing results on the DASH Diet varies from person to person. Some individuals may notice improvements in blood pressure within a few weeks, while others may take longer. Consistency with the DASH Diet principles and other lifestyle factors, such as regular physical activity, can influence the speed of results.

4. Is the DASH Diet Only for Those with High Blood Pressure?

- While the DASH Diet is renowned for its effectiveness in managing high blood pressure, it offers a well-rounded and heart-healthy approach suitable for anyone interested in promoting cardiovascular health. It can be beneficial for preventing hypertension, improving overall heart health, and supporting weight management.

5. Can I Use Salt Substitutes on the DASH Diet?

- Some individuals may choose to use salt substitutes, which often contain potassium chloride, as an alternative to traditional table salt. However, it's crucial to consult with a healthcare professional before incorporating salt substitutes, especially for those with kidney issues or taking medications that affect potassium levels.

6. Is It Challenging to Stick to the DASH Diet While Dining Out?

- While dining out may present challenges, it's entirely possible to make DASH-friendly choices. Look for grilled or roasted proteins, vegetable-based dishes, and whole grain options. Don't hesitate to request modifications, such as dressing on the side or substituting sides.

7. What If I Don't Enjoy Certain DASH-Recommended Foods?

- The DASH Diet offers flexibility, allowing you to choose from a variety of nutrient-dense foods. If there are specific foods you don't enjoy, explore alternative options within the same food group. For example, if you're not a fan of certain vegetables, try others that you find more appealing.

8. Can I Follow the DASH Diet as a Vegetarian or Vegan?

- Absolutely. The DASH Diet can be adapted to vegetarian or vegan lifestyles. Focus on plant-based protein sources, such as legumes, tofu, and tempeh, and incorporate a variety of fruits, vegetables, whole grains, and nuts. Ensure you get adequate nutrients like vitamin B12, iron, and omega-3 fatty acids through fortified foods or supplements.

9. Do I Need to Count Calories on the DASH Diet?

- The DASH Diet doesn't require strict calorie counting. Instead, it emphasizes portion control, choosing nutrient-dense foods, and making heart-healthy choices. Pay attention to hunger and fullness cues, and prioritize the quality of the foods you consume.

10. Can I Drink Alcohol on the DASH Diet?

- Moderate alcohol consumption is generally acceptable on the DASH Diet. However, it's essential to be mindful of portion sizes and choose drinks with lower added sugars. Men are advised to limit alcohol to two drinks per day, while women are recommended to limit to one drink per day.

12.2 Troubleshooting Meal Prep Challenges

1. I Find Meal Prep Overwhelming. How Can I Simplify the Process?

- Start small and gradually build your meal prep skills. Begin with basic recipes and simple meal plans. Consider prepping ingredients in advance, such as chopping vegetables or marinating proteins, to streamline the process.

2. I'm Bored with My Meal Options. How Can I Add Variety?

- Explore new recipes and cuisines to add excitement to your meals. Incorporate a diverse range of fruits, vegetables, whole grains, and proteins. Experiment with different herbs, spices, and cooking methods to enhance flavors.

3. I Don't Have Enough Time for Meal Prep. How Can I Make It More Efficient?

- Plan your meals and create a shopping list to streamline the process. Choose recipes with overlapping ingredients to minimize waste. Consider batch cooking on weekends and freezing portions for busy days.

4. My Family Members Have Different Dietary Preferences. How Can I Accommodate Everyone?

- Modify recipes to accommodate different preferences while still adhering to DASH Diet principles. For example, customize toppings or sides to suit individual tastes. Encourage open communication about dietary needs within the family.

5. I Struggle with Portion Control, Any Tips to Help?

- Use smaller plates to naturally control portion sizes. Be mindful of hunger and fullness cues, and avoid eating straight from containers. Pre-portion snacks and meals to prevent overeating.

6. I Often Forget to Prep Healthy Snacks, Any Suggestions?

- Plan snacks as part of your meal prep routine to ensure you have healthy options readily available. Pre-cut fruits and vegetables, portion nuts or seeds, and prepare yogurt parfaits for quick and nutritious snack choices.

7. My Meal Prep Doesn't Stay Fresh for the Whole Week. How Can I Improve Storage?

- Invest in quality food storage containers to maintain freshness. Store items like salads and dressings separately until ready to eat. Consider vacuum-sealing or using airtight containers for longer shelf life.

8. I Have Dietary Restrictions. How Can I Adapt DASH Diet Recipes?

- Modify recipes based on your dietary restrictions. Substitute ingredients as needed, and explore alternative options within the same food group. For personalized guidance, consult with a dietitian.

9. I Tend to Overeat When I'm Stressed. How Can I Address Emotional Eating?

- Identify alternative stress-management techniques, such as deep breathing, meditation, or engaging in a favorite hobby. Practice mindful eating by focusing on the sensory experience of each bite and recognizing emotional triggers.

10. I'm not seeing the Desired Results. What Might Be Going Wrong?

- Review your meal choices, portion sizes, and overall adherence to DASH Diet principles. Consider other lifestyle factors, such as physical activity and stress management. If results are not as expected, consult with a healthcare professional or dietitian for personalized guidance.

12.3 Seeking Professional Guidance

1. When Should I Consult with a Healthcare Professional or Dietitian?

- Consult with a healthcare professional or dietitian if you have pre-existing health conditions, are taking medications, or have specific dietary concerns. They can provide personalized advice based on your individual needs.

2. How Can a Dietitian Help Me on the DASH Diet?

- A dietitian can offer personalized guidance, create meal plans tailored to your preferences and dietary restrictions, and provide ongoing support. They can address specific health concerns, help with meal prep strategies, and optimize your nutrition for overall well-being.

3. What Should I Expect from a Healthcare Professional's Guidance?

- A healthcare professional can assess your overall health, review medical history, and offer guidance on managing specific health conditions. They may recommend lifestyle modifications, including dietary changes, to support your health goals.

4. Can a Healthcare Professional Help with Medication Adjustments?

- Healthcare professionals can assess the need for medication adjustments based on factors such as blood pressure readings and overall health. Any adjustments to medications should be made under their supervision.

5. Are Online Nutrition Programs Effective?

- Online nutrition programs can be effective, but the quality varies. Look for programs developed or endorsed by qualified professionals. Consider consulting with a dietitian for personalized guidance, especially if you have specific health concerns.

6. How Often Should I Follow Up with a Healthcare Professional or Dietitian?

- The frequency of follow-up depends on individual needs. For ongoing health management, regular follow-ups with a healthcare professional or dietitian can help track progress, make adjustments, and address any emerging concerns.

7. What Questions Should I Ask During a Consultation with a Healthcare Professional or Dietitian?

- Come prepared with questions about your specific health concerns, dietary preferences, and goals. Ask about recommended dietary changes, potential challenges, and strategies for long-term success.

8. Can I Trust Nutrition Information from Online Sources?

- While there is valuable nutrition information online, it's essential to rely on reputable sources. Look for information from registered dietitians, healthcare organizations, and academic institutions. Always cross-reference information to ensure accuracy.

9. What Role Does a Healthcare Professional Play in Monitoring Blood Pressure?

- A healthcare professional monitors blood pressure through regular measurements. They can interpret readings, assess overall cardiovascular health, and recommend lifestyle modifications or medications based on individual needs.

10. How Can I Advocate for My Dietary Preferences with Healthcare Professionals?

- Be open and transparent about your dietary preferences and concerns with healthcare professionals. Share your goals, any challenges you've faced, and your commitment to making positive changes. Collaborate with them to create a plan that aligns with your preferences and health needs

Remember that every person's experience is different as you plan your meals and follow the DASH Diet. Modify the tenets to fit your personal tastes, and don't be afraid to ask for expert advice when necessary. By addressing frequent issues, resolving difficulties with meal preparation, and taking into account expert assistance, you enable yourself to adopt a heart-healthy lifestyle that is consistent with your objectives and general well-being. To your ongoing success on the DASH Diet, cheers!

Chapter 13: Conclusion

Thank you for committing to a heart-healthy lifestyle and for reaching the final chapter of "The DASH DIET MEAL PREP: Delicious Heart-Healthy Recipes Low-Sodium, High-Potassium to Manage Blood Pressure." Your dedication to better health is truly admirable. We'll acknowledge your accomplishments, consider the DASH Diet's revolutionary potential, and discuss future heart-healthy lifestyle maintenance tactics in this last chapter.

13.1 Celebrating Your Journey to Better Health

Take a time to enjoy your trip as you consider the chapters you've read, the recipes you've tried, and the adjustments you've made. Every step you've taken toward improving your health, regardless of how long you've been following the DASH Diet, is a great step. Let's honor your accomplishments:

1. Embracing the DASH Diet Principles: Not only do you comprehend the DASH Diet's tenets, but you've also incorporated them into your regular activities. You've set yourself up for a heart-healthy lifestyle by putting an emphasis on fruits, vegetables, lean proteins, and whole grains while lowering your sodium consumption.

2. Mastering Meal Prep: You have become an expert at meal prep, from organizing your weekly menu to setting up your kitchen. The time and effort you've put into cooking scrumptious, wholesome meals is evidence of your dedication to long-term health.

3. Exploring Diverse Recipes: Through experimenting with the wide variety of dishes offered, you have broadened your culinary knowledge. You've elevated healthy eating to a beautiful experience, whether you're enjoying heart-healthy supper selections, nourishing salads, or revitalizing smoothie bowls.

4. Navigating Dining out Challenges: You've overcome the difficulties of eating out by making wise decisions that follow the DASH Diet. Your commitment to balance is demonstrated by your ability to enjoy social events while putting your heart health first.

5. Incorporating Physical Activity: It's excellent that you're incorporating exercise into your heart-healthy routine. Through regular walks, workouts, or leisure pursuits, you've adopted a comprehensive approach to overall health and wellness.

6. Managing Stress Effectively: By practicing mindfulness, deep breathing, and other stress-reduction methods, you've improved your mental and emotional health. Understanding the link between heart health and stress is an essential part of your journey.

7. Tracking Progress and Adjusting Your Plan: A growth mindset is demonstrated by your dedication to monitoring your success, making target adjustments, and maintaining an open mind. This flexibility is what will keep you moving forward on your heart-healthy journey.

8. Seeking Professional Guidance: By obtaining advice from medical professionals, dietitians, or seeking support for particular issues, you have exhibited a proactive approach to your well-being. Expert advice guarantees a comprehensive approach to heart health and supports your efforts.

9. Overcoming Meal Prep Challenges: Overcoming obstacles in meal preparation, such as time restraints or variety apprehensions, demonstrates your tenacity and will. Now that you've discovered solutions that work for you, meal planning is a fun and sustainable part of your daily routine.

10. Fostering a Positive Relationship with Food: Creating a healthy connection with food is essential to your path. Enjoy the satisfaction of providing your body with healthful, delectable meals and the awareness you bring to your eating routine.

11. Prioritizing Your Health: You've put your health and wellbeing first above anything else. Your dedication to developing a heart-healthy lifestyle is an investment that will pay off for the rest of your life in a world full of pressures.

Recognize the advancements you've made and the healthy routines you've adopted as you celebrate these successes. Keep in mind that improving your health is a continuous process, and each action you take will have an impact on your general health.

13.2 Forward-Looking: Maintaining a Heart-Healthy Way of Life

Now that you have established a solid basis for living a heart-healthy lifestyle, let's look at methods for maintaining and improving your wellbeing going forward:

1 Cultivate Mindful Eating Habits: By enjoying every bite, being aware of your body's signals of hunger and fullness, and relishing the flavors of your food, you can carry on your mindful eating practice. This thoughtful approach improves your entire dining experience and helps you develop a positive relationship with food.

2. Explore New Recipes and Flavors: Explore new flavors and recipes on a regular basis to keep your kitchen exciting. Try new cuisines, play around with ingredients, and push your cooking abilities. In addition to keeping meals engaging, variety guarantees a wide variety of nutrients.

3. Stay Active and Enjoy Movement: Include exercise on a regular basis in your regimen. Discover the joy of movement, whether it be via leisure activities, frequent walks, or workouts. To keep your exercise regimen interesting and pleasurable, think about attempting some new things.

4. Prioritize Quality Sleep: Maintain your focus on getting enough good sleep. A good night's sleep is crucial for maintaining general health and heart health in particular. For the best possible sleep, establish a relaxing evening ritual and make your surroundings conducive to relaxation.

5. Practice Stress Management: Make stress-reduction strategies a part of your everyday routine. Developing healthy coping mechanisms for stress, whether it is through mindfulness meditation, deep breathing techniques, or calming pastimes, enhances your general wellbeing.

6. Connect with a Support System: Keep up close relationships with loved ones who encourage you to pursue your health objectives. Rely on your network of support when things go tough, and share your journey and accomplishments with others. Emotional health is correlated with positive connections.

7. Regularly Monitor Your Blood Pressure: If controlling blood pressure is your specific objective, keep checking it on a regular basis. By taking the initiative, you may monitor your development, spot patterns, and, if necessary, modify your lifestyle plan with knowledge and insight.

8. Celebrate Milestones and Achievements: As you progress toward your health goals, set reasonable benchmarks and acknowledge your accomplishments. Acknowledging accomplishments encourages persistence in effort and reinforces positive behaviors.

9. Stay Informed and Open to Learning: Keep up with the most recent findings, dietary trends, and health advice. Making a commitment to lifelong learning gives you the ability to make decisions that support your health objectives.

10. Embrace Flexibility and Balance: Although maintaining a heart-healthy lifestyle requires consistency, accept flexibility. Because life is dynamic, changes could be required from time to time. React to changes with flexibility and a dedication to preserving equilibrium in every area of your life.

11. Inspire Others on Their Health Journey: Talk to people who could be traveling a similar path in terms of health about your experiences and learning. Your tale has the ability to uplift and encourage others, having a beneficial knock-on effect throughout your neighborhood.

12. Regularly Reassess Your Goals: Review your lifestyle and health objectives on a regular basis. Your priorities could change as things go on. Continue on your path to a sustainable future of well-being by modifying your goals to reflect your present aspirations.

13. Celebrate the Joy of Healthy Living: Accept the happiness that comes with leading a healthful life. Honor the vitality, vigor, and general state of health that come with living a heart-healthy lifestyle. Your dedication to taking care of yourself is a gift that keeps getting better.

Imagine a time when you will be vibrant, happy, and continue to be well. Making good decisions is a lifelong path towards improved health, and each one adds a unique color to your colorful life story. Keep in mind that you possess the resilience, knowledge, and abilities necessary to maintain a heart-healthy lifestyle that values your health and recognizes the amazing journey you've made.

Finally, I would like to thank you from the bottom of my heart for your commitment to improved health. May you have a heart that beats with the rhythm of a healthy, energetic existence, and may your days be full of tasty, nutritious food. Cheers to you, your well-being, and the incredible path that lies ahead!

About the Author

Dr. Adam C. stands as a beacon of inspiration in the fields of medicine, nutrition, and self-help, with a remarkable journey that exemplifies the transformative power of healthy living. Armed with a professional master's degree in health nutrition and years of experience, Dr. C. has become a guiding light for individuals seeking to embrace vibrant well-being and lead happier lives.

From an early age, Dr. C. navigated through a myriad of health challenges that ranged from genetic predispositions to the pitfalls of unhealthy eating. His personal struggle ignited a flame of determination within him, one that was fueled by the belief that the human body possesses an incredible ability to heal and rejuvenate through the right nourishment. Through steadfast dedication, Dr. C. managed to conquer his own ailments and emerged as a living testament to the transformative potential of a well-balanced lifestyle.

What sets Dr. Adam C. apart is his rich tapestry of experiences, having been deeply immersed in groundbreaking research in health food and diet-related domains. His quest to uncover the hidden treasures of nutrients within our meals has led to groundbreaking revel actions that empower individuals to extract the maximum benefit from their dietary choices. Dr. C.'s research has not only contributed to the scientific community but has also served as a roadmap for countless individuals striving to optimize their health.

However, it is not just Dr. C.'s academic prowess that has touched lives it is his unparalleled compassion and empathy that truly make him a beacon of hope. His personal journey of triumph over adversity infuses his guidance with an authentic understanding of the challenges his readers and patients face. Dr. C. doesn't just prescribe nutritional plans; he fosters a deep connection with his audience, instilling in them the confidence to embark on their own transformative journeys.

Dr. Adam C.'s holistic approach reaches beyond the confines of traditional medicine. His insights have translated into self-help resources that empower individuals to take charge of their wellness narrative. His words resonate on paper as they do in person, making his books not mere guides, but trusted companions on the path to vitality.

In the realm of health and nutrition, Dr. C. shines as a true luminary. His core strengths lie in his ability to synthesize complex scientific findings into practical, actionable advice that individuals from all walks of life can seamlessly integrate into their routines. Dr. C.'s legacy is not just a collection of breakthroughs; it is a testament to the extraordinary potential that lies within each of us to overcome obstacles and embrace a life brimming with health, happiness, and fulfillment.

As an experienced doctor, passionate nutritionist, and empathetic author, Dr. Adam C. continues to transform lives, showing us that the journey to a healthier, happier existence is within our grasp, waiting to be unlocked through the power of informed choices and unwavering determination.

www.ingramcontent.com/pod-product-compliance
Lightning Source LLC
Chambersburg PA
CBHW070902260726
48661CB00004B/1547

9 798887 290527